TATIANA FALCONE

A Parent's guide: to prevent suicide in your loved one

A tool for parents helping teens who are struggling with suicidality

First edition

This book was professionally typeset on Reedsy.
Find out more at reedsy.com

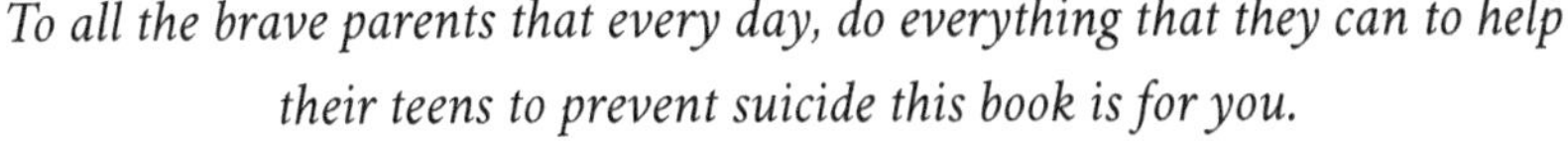

To all the brave parents that every day, do everything that they can to help
their teens to prevent suicide this book is for you.
To Michael, Camila and Sofi
and to the memory of Alexis Palencia

"You will one day experience joy that matches this pain. You will cry euphoric tears. You will stare down at a baby's face as she stare down in your lap. You will make great friends, you will try delicious foods. There are books that you haven't read, films you watch while eating popcorn. You will dance, and laugh and have sex… Life is waiting for you. You might be stuck here for a while, but the world isn't going anywhere. Hang on in there if you can. Life is always worth it"

Matt Haig

Contents

Foreword

Preface

1

Introduction

Why I am writing this book

I am a child and adolescent Psychiatrist, who is currently working at Cleveland Clinic for the last 22 years. Seventeen of those 22 years, I have been working specifically with parents and children. I divide my time between providing clinical care for youth with mental illness and doing research to improve the quality of life of youth and their families who struggle with mental illness. For the last 14 years, a bulk of my research has focused on suicide prevention, from the neurobiology of why youth become suicidal, to interventions (randomized control trials) on potential treatments to help suicidal teens anywhere from therapy to medication treatments.

I also have the privilege to work in a great hospital. Cleveland Clinic has been ranked the number 2 hospital in the world by Newsweek. (1) An on the best hospital honor roll for US News (2). One of our strengths is providing care for youth with chronic illnesses. I have been working closely with many providers of other specialties, who treat kids with chronic illness. I am part of the consultation team, who are called to see kids and their parents, probably in the worst moments of their lives.

After the kid is admitted to the hospital for a suicide attempt, or while in the hospital develop suicidal ideation or express any specific concern about self-harm.

Our psychiatry team spends countless hours every week, doing psycho education for parents on preventing suicide and 50% of my outpatient clinic consists of providing care to youth who are struggling with suicidal thoughts and their parents, or teens who were recently discharged from inpatient psychiatry after having a suicide attempt.

I am writing this book, as a resource guide for parents, to help support their teen and their family. To give you ideas of simple things that you can do at the moment to help your child. This book is not meant to replace acute care. If you or your loved one are in immediate need of help, please go to the nearest emergency room or call 988. By continuing to read this book, you acknowledge that it doesn't replace mental health care. Is always very important to take any suicide threats seriously and explore the need for urgent medical care by calling 988. This book is meant to be a resource tool for parents to navigate the complexity of helping their teen with suicidal thoughts. Always prioritize the safety of your teen, if you have worries about the current safety of your teen, please call 988. After you have taken the necessary steps to protect your teen, then please let's go back and continue reading this book.

2

Navigating Suicide Risk with Courageous Conversations

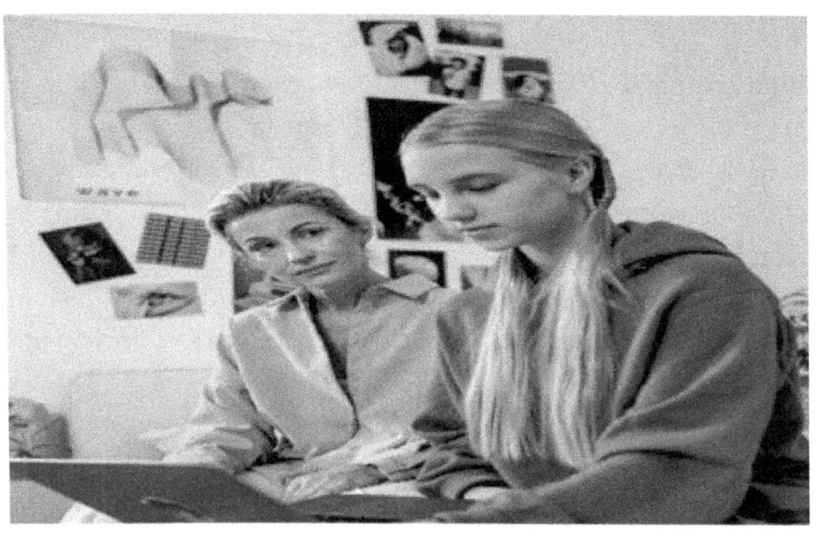

In the labyrinth of adolescence, where the sea of emotions collides with the search for identity, lies a silent struggle that demands our attention and compassion. It is within the hearts of our teens, amidst the turbulence of growth and self-discovery, that the shadows of suicide risk cast their somber silhouette.

In this chapter, we embark on a journey of vulnerability—a journey that invites us to explore the nuanced complexities of teen suicide risk through the lens of connection and compassion (3). Drawing inspiration from the wisdom of many parents like you who in moments like this felt the need to look for other things they could do to help their suicidal teen, we delve into the statistics, recognize warning signs, approach the topic with courage, challenge the impact of stigma, and debunk common myths surrounding suicide.

Illuminating the Statistics

In the landscape of teen suicide, statistics serve as a sobering reminder of the prevalence and urgency of the issue at hand. According to recent data, suicide remains one of the leading causes of death among adolescents worldwide. The numbers paint a stark picture—a picture that compels us to confront the harsh reality of teen suicide risk with courage and compassion (4).

Behind every statistic lies a story of anguish, despair, and unspoken pain. As we navigate the labyrinth of teen suicide, may we remember that each statistic represents a life—a life that is deserving of love, support, and understanding (4).

Recognizing Warning Signs

In the tapestry of teen suicide, warning signs emerge as silent whispers that beckon us to listen—to lean in with curiosity and compassion.

Helping suicidal teen requires that we become aware of their mental state and that we are opening a door to our hearts so we can listen to how they are feeling right now, without stigma, without blame, just listen not only to what they are saying but also how they are acting. Recognizing warning signs requires courage—the courage to see beyond the masks of adolescence and bear witness to the raw, unfiltered truth of our teens' experiences (4).

Warning signs may manifest in myriad forms—changes in behavior, mood swings, withdrawal from friends and activities, and expressions of hopelessness or despair. As trusted adults, parents, educators, and caregivers, it is our responsibility to remain vigilant—to create spaces where our teens feel seen, heard, and supported(7).

Approaching the Topic with Courage

In the realm of vulnerability, conversations about suicide demand our courage—the courage to lean into discomfort, to navigate the depths of despair with empathy and compassion(3). The most important step when you approach this topic is to check your internal pulse, meaning that we know is scary to talk about suicide, understand your feelings before you approach the conversation, and make sure that you make your teen feel heard, supported, let them open their heart no matter how hard might before you as a parent to hear those words. Approaching the topic of suicide requires authenticity—the willingness to engage with our teens in open, honest dialogue without judgment or shame(3).

As we embark on these courageous conversations, may we remember that our presence is the greatest gift we can offer—a beacon of hope a midst the darkness, a lifeline of connection in times of despair. In the tender embrace of vulnerability, may our words be imbued with kindness, empathy, and unwavering support(3).

The Impact of Stigma

In the shadows of suicide risk, stigma lurks as the silent specter that perpetuates shame and silence. Stigma thrives in the absence of empathy and understanding—in the darkness where fear and ignorance hold sway. To challenge the impact of stigma, we must confront our own biases, cultivate empathy, and create spaces where vulnerability is met with compassion rather than judgment(4).

Stigma erects barriers to help-seeking behavior, perpetuating the myth that vulnerability is synonymous with weakness. As allies in the fight against stigma, may we stand in solidarity with our teens, offering support, understanding, and unconditional acceptance. For your teen to feel confident that they can trust you no matter how hard the conversation is, they have to see and feel that when they come to you in the moment of need, you will embrace them and support them without casting any shame or guilt, just unconditional love. They have to feel the radical acceptance, that you are there for them no matter what, and that you won't judge them, just protect them and love them (4).

Debunking Common Myths Regarding Suicide

Myths surrounding suicide weave a tangled web of misinformation and misunderstanding. Debunking these myths requires courage—the courage to challenge societal norms, confront misconceptions, and embrace the truth with openness and humility.

Contrary to popular belief, suicide is not a choice—it is a manifestation of unrelenting pain and despair. By debunking common myths surrounding suicide, we pave the way for healing, understanding, and authentic connection.

In the realm of adolescent mental health, misinformation often shrouds the conversation surrounding suicide. Marsha Linehan, renowned for her pioneering work in dialectical behavior therapy, emphasizes the importance of dispelling common myths to foster understanding and promote effective intervention.

Myth: Talking about suicide will plant the idea in a teen's mind.

Reality: Contrary to this belief, open dialogue about suicide does not induce suicidal thoughts. It can create a safe space for teens to express their emotions and seek help when needed. Acknowledging their struggles validates their experiences and encourages them to reach out for support(7).

Myth: Teens who talk about suicide are just seeking attention and won't actually follow through.

Reality: Every expression of suicidal ideation deserves attention and intervention. Dismissing these cries for help as mere attention-seeking behavior undermines the severity of their emotional distress. It is crucial to take all discussions of suicide seriously and provide compassionate support and resources (4).

Myth: Teens who attempt suicide are weak or selfish.

Reality: Suicide attempts stem from immense emotional pain and turmoil, not weakness or selfishness. Adolescents facing suicidal thoughts often feel overwhelmed by their circumstances and see suicide as the only means of escape. Understanding the depth of their suffering is essential in offering them the support and validation they desperately need (4).

Myth: Once a teen exhibits suicidal behavior, there's nothing anyone can do to help.

Reality: Intervention and support can make a significant difference in preventing suicide. With appropriate therapy, support networks, and access to mental health resources, teens can find hope and healing. By addressing the underlying issues contributing to their distress, we can empower them to navigate their challenges and build resilience (7).

By debunking these myths, we can foster empathy, understanding, and effective intervention, ultimately saving lives and promoting mental well-being. In the tender terrain of teen suicide, may we approach the topic of suicide with courage, empathy, and unwavering support. In the quiet corners of our hearts, may we hold space for our teens' struggles, fears, and unspoken pain. And in the embrace of vulnerability, may we find the courage to navigate the labyrinth of adolescence with compassion, understanding, and unwavering love.

3

Understanding Teen Suicide: Unraveling the Complexities with Compassion and Insight

In the intricate tapestry of adolescent mental health, the specter of suicide casts a long shadow—a silent testament to the profound struggles that teens face in navigating the tumultuous terrain of adolescence. Let us explore the multifaceted factors that may contribute to a teen's decision to attempt suicide with empathy, understanding, and unwavering compassion.

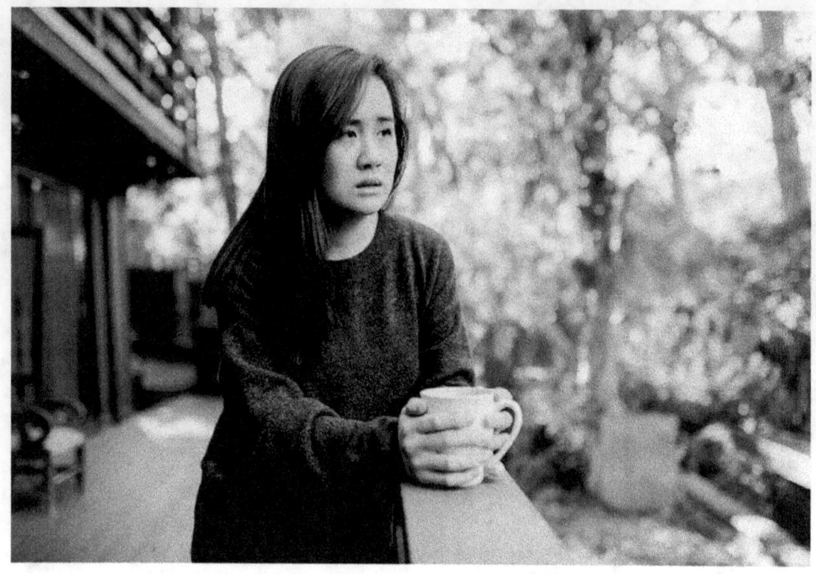

Stress: Navigating the Pressure Cooker of Adolescence

For many teens, the weight of academic expectations, peer pressure, and familial responsibilities can become an overwhelming burden. In the pressure cooker of adolescence, stress mounts like a simmering cauldron, threatening to boil over at any moment. It is important to understand that even though stress is a natural part of life, excessive and unrelenting stress can tip the scales, plunging teens into a state of emotional turmoil and despair.

In the landscape of adolescent mental health, stress emerges as a formidable driver for suicide—a silent yet pervasive force that exerts its grip on the hearts and minds of young individuals. As described by Dr. Jobes in the CAMS framework, stress has a critical role in shaping the trajectory of suicidal thoughts and behaviors among adolescents (7).

For many teens, the pressures of academic expectations, social dynamics, and familial responsibilities create a crucible of stress that threatens to overwhelm their fragile sense of well-being. Jobes highlights that stress is not simply a transient inconvenience but a profound disruptor of emotional equilibrium, fueling feelings of hopelessness and despair (7).

In moments of stress, adolescents may find themselves navigating a labyrinth of uncertainty and turmoil, grappling with the weight of expectations and the fear of failure. Chronic stress erodes the resilience of young minds, leaving them vulnerable to the insidious whispers of suicidal ideation (4).

The relentless onslaught of stressors can shatter the protective barriers that shield adolescents from the depths of despair, leaving them adrift in a sea of emotional turmoil. It is so very important for parents to recognize the warning signs of stress-induced distress and intervene proactively to mitigate the risk of suicide.

Understanding stress as a driver for suicide in adolescents requires a multifaceted approach that addresses the underlying sources of distress while fostering resilience and coping skills. Jobes advocates for comprehensive suicide prevention strategies that prioritize early intervention, destigmatize help-seeking behaviors, and promote a culture of open communication and support. By addressing the root causes of stress and providing adolescents with the resources they need to navigate life's challenges, we can offer hope and healing in the face of adversity. As a parent providing company, support, and distraction in those moments of high stress in teens can be very valuable.

Hopelessness: The Absence of Light in the Darkness

In the darkest depths of despair, hopelessness looms as a suffocating fog, enveloping teens in its oppressive embrace. Marsha Linehan underscores that hopelessness is not merely a fleeting emotion but a pervasive sense of futility and despair—a belief that there is no escape from the pain and suffering that grips their hearts. In the absence of hope, the prospect of suicide may appear as the only means of relief from the relentless agony of their existence (4).

For many teens, hopelessness is not simply a passing emotion but a profound sense of despair—a belief that their circumstances will never improve, and their pain will never subside. Hopelessness is not a sign of weakness or moral failure but a natural response to overwhelming adversity and emotional distress.

In the depths of hopelessness, teens may feel trapped in a suffocating wave of despair, unable to envision a future beyond the pain that consumes them. The relentless whispers of self-doubt and despair echo in the corridors of their minds, drowning out any flicker of hope that dares to ignite.

Understanding hopelessness requires us to bear witness to the depths of teen despair—to hold space for their pain and validate their experiences without judgment or condemnation. By acknowledging the profound impact of hopelessness on teen mental health, we can offer them the compassion, understanding, and support they need to navigate the stormy seas of adolescence and rediscover the glimmer of hope that lies within. Helping teens build hope one day at a time, is perhaps one of the most important interventions that any parent can do to help their teen to create a life worth living(4).

Emotional Pain: The Unseen Wounds of the Soul

Beneath the facade of adolescent bravery lies a wellspring of emotional pain—an invisible burden that weighs heavily on the hearts of teens. Emotional pain, though intangible, can inflict wounds as profound as any physical injury. Whether stemming from trauma, loss, or internal struggles, the anguish of emotional pain can erode the resilience of even the strongest spirits, leaving teens feeling utterly shattered and alone(7).

In 2015, we conducted a study comparing adolescents admitted to inpatient psychiatry who had experienced different kinds of emotional trauma and at the moment currently experiencing suicidal thoughts with healthy adolescents, we used several biological markers in both populations. One of the biomarkers we used was the protein S100B, a protein that has been used in other studies to evaluate the impact of brain trauma. We were surprised to learn that adolescents with suicidal thoughts, had really high levels of this protein, and those who experienced more severe, chronic, and early trauma (before age 8 years old), were more likely to have suicidal thoughts. Also, the impact of emotional trauma was as severe as the impact of traumatic brain injury as measured by the S100B protein(5).

Agitation: The Storm Within

In the tempest of adolescence, agitation swirls like a turbulent storm, threatening to consume teens in its tumultuous wake. Agitation is not simply restlessness or irritability but a manifestation of inner turmoil— a relentless whirlwind of thoughts and emotions that rages unchecked within their minds. Unable to find respite, teens may see suicide as a desperate attempt to quiet the storm and find peace amid chaos.

In the realm of suicide prevention, understanding agitation as a potent driver for suicidal thoughts is paramount. Several authors have shed light on the profound impact of agitation on individuals grappling with suicidal ideation(7).

Agitation, characterized by restlessness, irritability, and an overwhelming sense of unease, serves as a turbulent undercurrent that propels individuals toward the precipice of despair. Jobes emphasizes that agitation is not merely a transient state of discomfort but a powerful force that exacerbates the intensity of suicidal thoughts and impulses(10).

For those experiencing agitation, the relentless onslaught of racing thoughts and overwhelming emotions can become unbearable. Agitation amplifies feelings of hopelessness and despair, eroding the individual's capacity to cope with life's challenges and envision a future free from pain.

In the throes of agitation, individuals may feel trapped in a relentless cycle of turmoil, desperately seeking respite from the relentless storm raging within. In his innovative third edition of the CAMS framework, Jobes identifies how agitation catalyzes impulsive and reckless behaviors, further heightening the risk of self-harm and suicide.

Understanding agitation as a driver for suicidal thoughts requires a nuanced and compassionate approach to suicide prevention. Jobes advocates for comprehensive risk assessment protocols that prioritize the identification and management of agitation as a critical component of suicide risk. By addressing the underlying factors contributing to agitation and providing targeted interventions aimed at restoring a sense of calm and stability, parents can offer hope and support to individuals navigating the turbulent waters of suicidal ideation (7).

Self-Esteem: The Fragile Mirror of Self-Worth

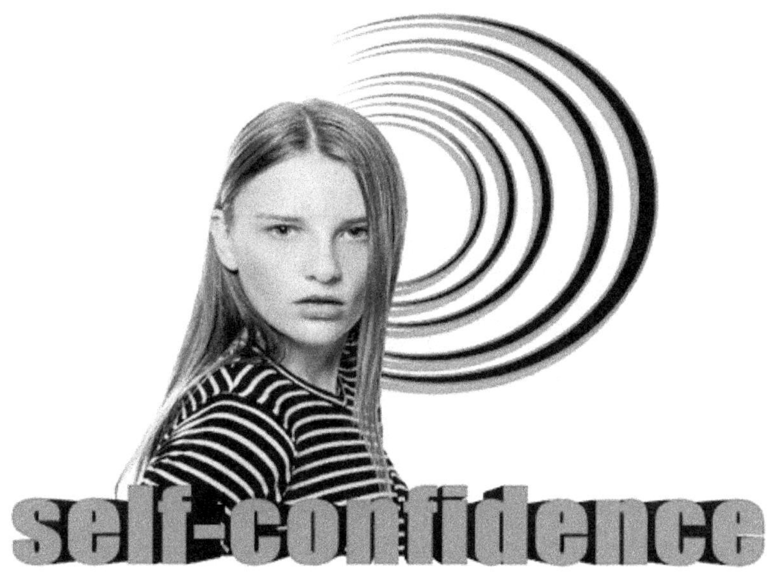

In the mirror of self-esteem, teens may see distorted reflections of their worth and value—a fractured image distorted by the harsh judgments of others and the relentless voice of self-doubt. Marsha Linehan teaches us that low self-esteem is not a reflection of inherent inadequacy but a product of societal pressures, unrealistic expectations, and internalized beliefs of unworthiness. In the absence of self-love and acceptance, teens may see suicide as a final, desperate attempt to escape the suffocating grip of their own perceived shortcomings. Anything that we can do as parents to foster the improvement of teens' self-esteem, such as creating opportunities for discoveries of new talents (new hobbies), and finding and pointing to your teen some of their inner strengths, can be really helpful. When someone is struggling with depression they struggle to recognize the positive, having you as a mirror that can help them see some of the positive in their life, the time when they are struggling with suicidal thoughts, could be lifesaving(4).

The Role of Mental Illness: Unraveling the Threads of Complexity

In the labyrinth of teen suicide, mental illness emerges as a tangled web of complexity—a pervasive force that colors perceptions, distorts reality, and robs teens of their sense of self. Mental illness is not a character flaw or a sign of weakness but a medical condition that requires understanding, compassion, and effective treatment. Mental illness is like any other medical illness, you wouldn't ask someone who just broke their leg to hope patiently until everything gets better, you will take them to the appropriate care to make sure they get the care they need to fix the broken leg, is the same for mental illness. Whether grappling with depression, anxiety, or other psychiatric disorders, teens may find themselves ensnared in a web of despair from which suicide seems like the only escape. There is effective treatment in the form of medication and/ or therapy that can help improve the symptoms of mental illness, and improve the quality of life of those suffering from it(7-11).

Grief and Other Losses: Navigating the Shadows of Sorrow

In the aftermath of loss, grief casts a long shadow—a silent testament to the depth of love and the pain of separation. Grief is not a linear journey but a complex tapestry of emotions—anger, sadness, guilt, and longing— that waxes and wanes like the tides of the sea. Whether mourning the loss of a loved one, a cherished dream, or a sense of security, teens may find themselves adrift in a sea of sorrow, seeking solace in the darkness of suicide's embrace(12).

In the realm of adolescent mental health, the intersection of suicide and grief emerges as an important one—a testament to the profound impact of loss on young hearts and minds. Let's explore the topic of grief with compassion and understanding. The way how adolescents perceive grief might be somewhat different and at times hard to understand from the parents' point of view.

For teens grappling with the aftermath of a peer's suicide, grief takes on myriad forms—anger, sadness, confusion, and profound disbelief. Suicide-related grief is not a linear journey but a meandering path marked by twists and turns, highs and lows. As parents is important to take into account, how important anniversaries will bring some of the memories and feelings back, to plan and be emotionally and physically available when this happens(13).

When exploring adolescent grief, teens may find themselves adrift in a sea of unanswered questions and unspoken pain. Wolfelt emphasizes the importance of creating safe spaces where teens can express their emotions openly and without judgment, offering them the validation and support they need to navigate the complexities of their grief journey(26).

Understanding suicide-related grief in teens requires a compassionate and nuanced approach—one that acknowledges the unique challenges and vulnerabilities they face in the aftermath of loss. Wolfelt advocates for community-based support networks that provide teens with the resources and guidance they need to process their grief and find healing amid despair. By embracing the principles of empathy, understanding, and unconditional love, we can offer support to grieving teens as they navigate the loss and find hope in sorrow(26).

Trauma: The Lingering Echoes of Pain

In the wake of trauma, the echoes of pain reverberate through the corridors of the mind—a haunting reminder of past wounds that refuse to heal. Marsha Linehan emphasizes that trauma is not simply a singular event but a pervasive force that can shatter the very foundations of a teen's sense of safety and security. Whether grappling with the aftermath of abuse, neglect, or violence, teens may find themselves trapped in a cycle of fear and despair, seeking escape from the finality of suicide(4).

Understanding teen suicide requires us to explore the intricate interplay of stress, hopelessness, emotional pain, agitation, self-esteem, mental illness, grief, and trauma with empathy and insight. By shining a light into the darkness of adolescent despair, we can offer teens the compassion, understanding, and support they need to find hope, healing, and a reason to choose life(17).

In the intricate tapestry of adolescent mental health, trauma emerges as a profound and often overlooked driver for suicide—a silent yet formidable force that casts a long shadow over the lives of young individuals. For many teens, the specter of trauma lurks in the shadows of their past—a haunting reminder of experiences that have left indelible scars on their hearts and minds. Haig emphasizes that trauma is not merely a singular event but a pervasive force that can shape the very fabric of a teen's identity, leaving them vulnerable to suicide.

In the aftermath of trauma, teens may find themselves grappling with a myriad of emotions—fear, anger, shame, and profound despair. Trauma disrupts the delicate balance of the adolescent psyche, robbing teens of their sense of safety and security in the world. It affects how teens perceive the world and how they react to stress now, in some cases making them unable to cope with stressors that for other people who have not experienced traumatic experiences might seem simple. As parents, is very important to check how are we reacting when the teen is experiencing these feelings, making sure that we are supportive, engaged, and anchored to what is happening at the moment, remember people who have experienced trauma, might be mentally stuck on prior experiences, one of the important roles of parents is helping the teen found grounding techniques that can bring them back to the actual moment(4).

The lingering echoes of trauma can cast a long shadow over the lives of young individuals, fueling feelings of hopelessness and worthlessness. Haig highlights the importance of creating safe and nurturing environments where teens feel empowered to share their experiences and seek support without fear of judgment or stigma.

Understanding the complex interplay between trauma and suicide in teens requires a compassionate and holistic approach. Haig advocates for trauma-informed care that prioritizes empathy, understanding, and validation, offering teens the tools and resources they need to heal from their past wounds and reclaim their sense of agency and purpose in life. By shining a light into the darkness of trauma, we can offer hope and healing to teens as they navigate the turbulent waters of adolescence (18-21).

4

Navigating an Acute Suicide Crisis: Empowering Teens with Compassion and Support

If you have acute concerns about the safety of your teen now, please take them to the Emergency room or call 988. Tomorrow might be too late.

Supporting Teens in an Acute Suicide Crisis

When faced with an acute suicide crisis, it is essential to respond with compassion and urgency. When a teen is acutely suicidal, is a medical emergency, like having appendicitis, you have to act now and make sure first that they are safe in the moment. It is very important to validate teens' experiences and offer a safe space for them to express their emotions without judgment. Encouraging open communication and active listening can help teens feel heard, understood, and supported during times of crisis (18).

It is crucial to assess the immediate risk of harm and take appropriate action to ensure the teen's safety. This may involve removing access to lethal means, such as medications or firearms, and connecting the teen with mental health professionals or crisis intervention services (20).

Offering practical support, such as helping the teen develop a safety plan or identifying coping strategies, can empower them to navigate the crisis and build resilience in the face of adversity. By fostering a sense of hope and agency, we can help teens find the strength to weather the storm and emerge stronger on the other side. Parents play a critical role in safeguarding their teens' well-being during times of acute crisis.

First and foremost, parents must remain calm and composed, providing a stable and supportive presence for their teen in crisis. Actively listening to their teen's concerns without judgment or criticism, creating a safe space for open and honest communication. Parents should take all expressions of suicidal ideation seriously, recognizing them as cries for help rather than mere attention-seeking behavior. Validating their teen's emotions and experiences, acknowledging the depth of their pain and despair without minimizing or dismissing their struggles. A good rule to help people feel heard is that you validate every feeling at least 3 times, so your teen can feel that you are listening to them. Is very important that during an acute suicide crisis, your teen is not left alone (19).

Above all, parents must convey unconditional love and support to their teens, reassuring them that they are not alone in their struggles and that help is available. By fostering a sense of trust and belonging, parents can empower their teens to seek the help they need and embark on the journey of healing and recovery.

Helping Teens Cope with Acute Suicidal Thoughts

When supporting a teen coping with acute suicidal thoughts, it is essential to approach the situation with empathy and understanding. Radical acceptance, support without judgment, the importance of acknowledging the depth of the teen's pain, and again validating their emotions without minimizing or dismissing their experiences(4).

Encouraging teens to explore the underlying triggers and contributors to their suicidal thoughts can help them gain insight into their emotional distress and identify healthier coping mechanisms. Providing them with tools and resources, such as crisis hotlines (988), support groups, and therapy options, can offer a lifeline of support during times of crisis. Promoting a sense of connection and belonging can also help teens feel less isolated and alone in their struggles. Encouraging them to reach out to trusted friends, family members, or mental health professionals can foster a supportive network of individuals who are invested in their well-being (18).

Assisting Teens in Coping with Depressive Symptoms

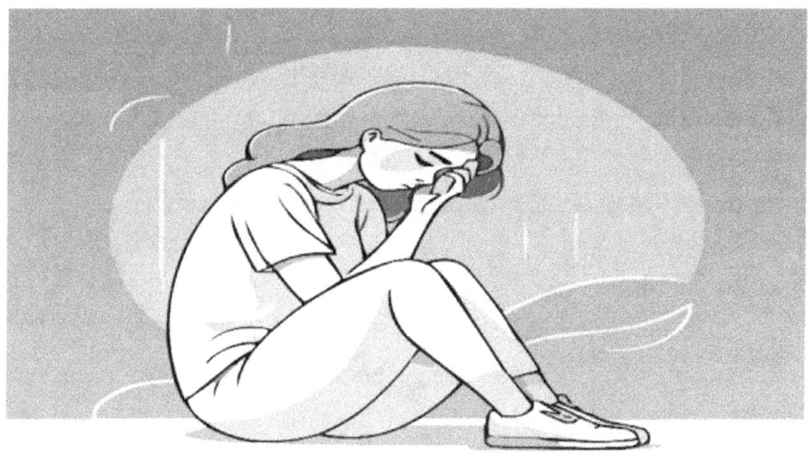

Depressive symptoms can severely impact the lives of teens, making it challenging to find joy or hope amid despair. Depression is a medical illness, there are effective treatments (medication and/or therapy) that can potentially improve the symptoms. A multifaceted approach to helping teens cope with depressive symptoms is encouraged addressing both the emotional and practical aspects of their struggles.

Encouraging teens to engage in activities that bring them pleasure and fulfillment can help alleviate feelings of sadness and hopelessness. Whether it's spending time outdoors, pursuing creative interests, or connecting with supportive peers, finding moments of joy can be a powerful antidote to depression.

Teaching teens mindfulness and relaxation techniques, such as deep breathing exercises or guided imagery, can help them manage stress and anxiety more effectively. By cultivating a sense of mindfulness, teens can learn to observe their thoughts and emotions without judgment, fostering greater self-awareness and emotional resilience.

We encourage teens who are struggling with depression, to engage in daily activities even if they don't feel they want to, the more isolated and disengaged the teen becomes, the worse the depressive symptoms, and the higher the risk for suicidal thoughts to come back(4,8-9).

Supporting Teens in Coping with Anxiety Symptoms

Anxiety symptoms can be debilitating, causing teens to feel overwhelmed and paralyzed by fear. Is important to help teens develop healthy coping strategies to manage their anxiety and regain a sense of control over their lives.

Encouraging teens to practice grounding techniques, such as focusing on their breathing or engaging in sensory activities, can help alleviate feelings of panic and distress. By grounding themselves in the present moment, teens can disrupt the cycle of anxious thoughts and regain a sense of calm and stability.

Promoting healthy lifestyle habits, such as regular exercise, nutritious eating, and adequate sleep, can also play a crucial role in managing anxiety symptoms. By taking care of their physical health, teens can enhance their resilience to stress and improve their overall well-being(18).

Encouraging teens to challenge negative thought patterns and replace them with more balanced and realistic perspectives can help reduce anxiety and increase feelings of self-efficacy. By re framing their thoughts, teens can learn to approach challenges with greater confidence and resilience.

If our goal is to help teens navigate acute suicidal thoughts, depressive symptoms, and anxiety requires a compassionate, cooperative, and holistic approach.First, we should learn to recognize the symptoms of anxiety and depression in our teens. Then create the opportunity for fostering connection, validating emotions, and empowering teens to find hope and resilience in the face of adversity. By offering unwavering support and understanding, we can help teens weather the storms of adolescence and emerge stronger, more resilient, and more hopeful for the future.

5

Supporting Individuals with Chronic Suicidal Thoughts: Navigating the Path to Healing with Compassion

When helping a teen with chronic suicidal thoughts, compassion becomes the guiding light—of hope that illuminates the path to healing and recovery(3).

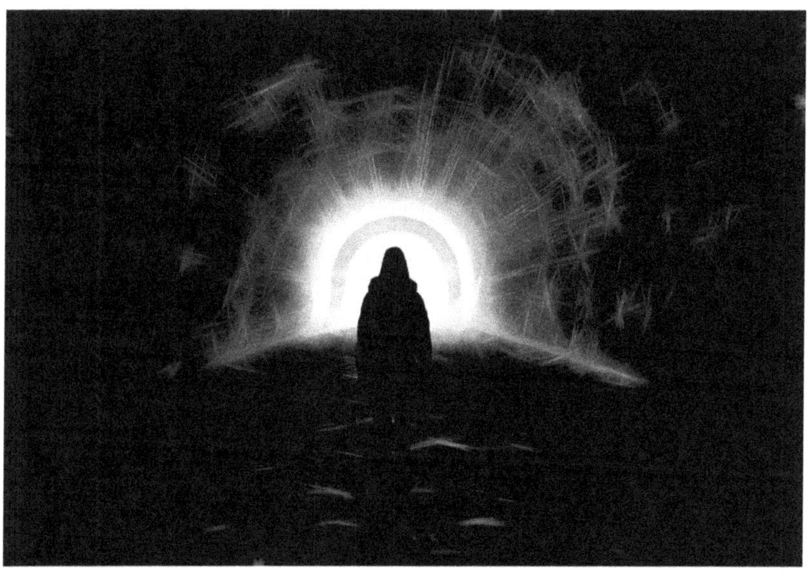

Assessing the Kind of Help They Need Now

In the intricate landscape of chronic suicidal thoughts, the first step in offering support is to assess the individual's immediate needs with compassion and empathy. It is very important to create a safe and non-judgmental space where individuals feel comfortable expressing their emotions and sharing their struggles (4).

Assessing the kind of help they need now requires a holistic approach—one that considers their unique experiences, challenges, and strengths. It is essential to listen actively (with all of our senses) and validate their emotions, acknowledging the depth of their pain and despair without minimizing or dismissing their struggles (4).

Encouraging open communication and collaboration can help individuals feel empowered to take an active role in their recovery journey. By engaging in a collaborative dialogue, we can gain insight into their needs and preferences, tailoring our support to align with their goals and aspirations (7).

How to Be Supportive to Someone with Chronic Suicidality

Being supportive of someone with chronic suicidality requires a multifaceted approach—one that encompasses empathy, validation, and practical assistance. Again validating their emotions and experiences, acknowledging the depth of their pain and despair without judgment or criticism (4).

Offering a compassionate presence and active listening can provide individuals with a sense of comfort and reassurance, fostering a deeper connection and trust. It is essential to convey empathy and understanding, validating their struggles, and offering hope for a brighter tomorrow. Helping them identify what are some of the goals that can bring a brighter tomorrow, helping them see the possibility of the future, while also making them feel an important part of the family (one that has roles and responsibilities) (4).

Practical assistance, such as helping them develop coping skills and safety plans, can empower individuals to navigate moments of crisis with greater resilience and self-efficacy. Dialectical Behavioral Therapy (DBT) is one of the therapies that has been identified as an evidence-based practice to improve chronic suicidality, focusing on certain tools, such as mindfulness, distress tolerance, emotion regulation, and interpersonal effectiveness, to help individuals build healthier coping mechanisms and enhance their overall well-being (8).

Encouraging individuals to engage in self-care activities that promote relaxation and stress reduction can also play a crucial role in managing chronic suicidal thoughts. Whether it's practicing mindfulness, engaging in physical activity, or pursuing creative outlets, finding moments of joy and fulfillment can provide individuals with a sense of purpose and meaning a midst their struggles (8).

Above all, being supportive of someone with chronic suicidality requires patience, empathy, and unwavering commitment. Healing is a journey—a journey marked by setbacks and triumphs, but ultimately leading toward a place of hope and resilience. By offering unconditional support and understanding, we can walk alongside individuals in their darkest moments and help them find the strength to embrace life with courage and determination (8).

6

The Invisible Struggle: Chronic Illness and Suicidal Teens

Chronic illness emerges as a silent specter—a formidable adversary that casts a long shadow over the lives of young individuals.

Unraveling the Complexity of Chronic Illness

At the heart of the issue lies the profound impact of chronic illness on the physical, emotional, and psychological well-being of teens. Epilepsy, diabetes, chronic pain, cancer, PTSD, migraines, and the recent emergence of COVID-19 have reshaped the landscape of adolescent health, challenging the resilience and fortitude of young individuals in unforeseen ways(38).

The Invisible Struggle: Unmasking Suicidal Ideation

Beneath the veneer of resilience lies the invisible struggle of teens coping with chronic illness—a struggle that often goes unnoticed and unaddressed. The relentless demands of chronic illness, navigating a labyrinth of physical discomfort, emotional distress, and existential uncertainty

Epilepsy: Seizing Control of the Unknown

For teens living with epilepsy, each seizure serves as a stark reminder of the unpredictability of their condition—a reminder that life hangs in the balance between moments of clarity and convulsions. There is an important psychological toll of epilepsy, highlighting the sense of powerlessness and vulnerability that often accompanies the condition (29-31).

Children with epilepsy are at higher risk of suffering from depression; the lifetime prevalence is reported up to 50% in some studies. Access to treatment in children with special health care needs in some cases might be worse than in the general population, putting these patients at risk for suicide . The incidence of depression in children with epilepsy varies between 25%-35% compared to 1- 2% in healthy pre-pubertal children and 3-8% in adolescents (23-24). The mental health needs of children with epilepsy are largely unmet, contributing to longer periods of depression that may continue through adulthood (29) Patients with epilepsy and depression have some of the lowest scores on quality-of-life scales, even when seizures are under control

In a study that we conducted using big data from open-source conversations of people with epilepsy 222 000 unique conversations were identified in 1 year in the US, and 4% of those (9000) were about suicide, we also identified that teenagers with epilepsy engage in online conversations more than adults with epilepsy (34).

Diabetes: The Sweet Burden of Management

In the world of diabetes, teens find themselves walking a tightrope between strict dietary restrictions and fluctuating blood sugar levels—a delicate balancing act that demands unwavering vigilance and discipline. Studies report the psychological impact of diabetes, revealing the pervasive sense of isolation and frustration that can accompany the daily management of the condition. Studies have reported that suicidal thoughts in youth with type 1 diabetes are frequent, in some studies the incidence could be as high as 15% (35-36).

Chronic Pain: The Silent Agony of Adolescence

In the shadow of chronic pain, teens grapple with a relentless torment that defies explanation—a torment that seeps into every aspect of their lives, leaving no refuge from the unrelenting agony. Teens experiencing chronic pain, as well as adults are at higher risk of suicide. Perhaps the profound sense of hopelessness and despair that can envelop teens in its suffocating embrace.

For teens struggling with chronic pain, each day becomes a relentless battle against an invisible adversary—a battle marked by physical discomfort, emotional distress, and existential uncertainty. Chronic pain is not merely a physical sensation but a pervasive force that permeates every aspect of a teen's life, robbing them of their sense of normalcy and well-being. When the pain is hard to control teens might find themselves with feelings of despair, hopelessness, isolation, frustration, and helplessness.

The relentless torment of chronic pain can erode a teen's resilience and diminish their sense of purpose and meaning in life. Without proper support and intervention, teens may become overwhelmed by their pain and see suicide as the only means of escape from their suffering.

Understanding the link between chronic pain and suicide in teens requires a compassionate and multidimensional approach—one that addresses the physical, emotional, and psychological dimensions of their pain. Management of chronic pain is a critical component of suicide prevention.

By offering teens the support, validation, and resources they need to cope with their chronic pain, we can help them find hope and resilience in the face of adversity. With empathy and understanding, we can empower teens to navigate their pain and reclaim their lives with courage and determination (37).

Cancer: Navigating the Uncertainty of Survival

For teens facing the daunting prospect of cancer, each day becomes a battle against the unknown—a battle marked by fear, uncertainty, and the constant specter of mortality. In a study of more than 50,000 youth with cancer, the risk of suicidal thoughts was reported to be 2.3 times higher than in the general population, the risk in women was 4 times higher than in men. Coping with side effects from medication as well as uncertainty can certainly impact hope and be one of the drivers of suicidal thoughts in youth with cancer (38).

PTSD: The Lingering Echoes of Trauma

In the complex realm of adolescent mental health, post-traumatic stress disorder (PTSD) emerges as a poignant contributor to suicidal ideation among teens. The profound impact of traumatic experiences can cast a long shadow over the lives of young individuals, leaving them vulnerable to the insidious whispers of despair and hopelessness.

Teens grappling with PTSD often find themselves in a web of intrusive memories, flashbacks, and nightmares—a web that threatens to engulf them in a vortex of emotional turmoil and despair. The relentless onslaught of traumatic reminders can erode their sense of safety and security, leaving them full of uncertainty and fear.

The psychological scars of PTSD run deep, leaving teens feeling disconnected from themselves and the world around them. The pervasive sense of numbness and detachment can exacerbate feelings of isolation and alienation, further isolating teens from the support and connection they desperately need.

When coping with PTSD, teens may find themselves grappling with overwhelming emotions—anger, sadness, guilt, and shame—that threaten to consume them from within. The invisible wounds of trauma can leave teens feeling powerless and alone, with suicide seeming like the only escape from their pain and suffering.

Understanding the link between PTSD and suicide in teens requires a compassionate and holistic approach. By offering teens the support, validation, and resources they need to navigate their trauma, we can help them find hope and healing when dealing with despair. With empathy and understanding, we can empower teens to reclaim their lives and rewrite their stories with courage and resilience (17-20).

COVID-19: The Unseen Enemy

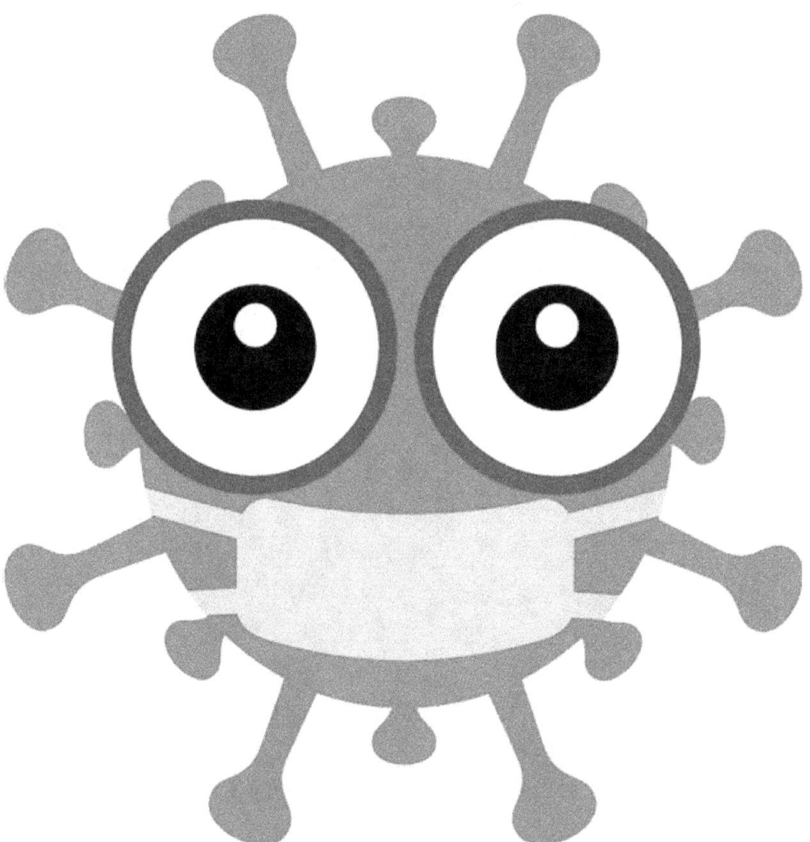

In the wake of the COVID-19 pandemic, teens find themselves grappling with a new and unfamiliar threat—one that has reshaped their world and irrevocably altered the course of their lives.The psychological impact of COVID-19, reveals the pervasive sense of fear, uncertainty, and isolation that can accompany the pandemic. We have observed an increase in reports of suicidal ideation and behaviors, especially in the first year of the COVID-19 pandemic, in youth and also in youth with chronic illness, our study focused in youth with epilepsy, vs. youth with no chronic illness. We reviewed well child and sick visits between Jan 1st of 2020 and Sep of 2020, during this period we have screening questionnaires from 21,134 youth who came to see the pediatrician. The scores were significant for depression in 4% of the youth (905 patients). 10% endorsed some level of feeling they would be better off dead or having thoughts of hurting themselves in some way, and 4.3% endorsed having serious thoughts about ending their life in the past month. We saw some variation in the months in which patients reported suicidal thoughts, being worse during the months of the stay-at-home order.(46)

7

Understanding Suicide Risk in Teen Populations: Navigating the Intersection of Mental Health and Vulnerability

I n the enigmatic landscape of adolescent mental health, certain populations of teens find themselves at higher risk for suicide—a stark reminder of the intricate interplay between psychological distress and vulnerability. Let's explore how certain conditions predispose teens to a higher risk of suicide.

Depression and Suicide

Depression emerges as a potent precursor to suicide among teens. emphasizes that the pervasive feelings of hopelessness, worthlessness, and despair that accompany depression can render teens particularly vulnerable to suicidal thoughts and behaviors. The worse the depression becomes, the higher the risk of suicide. Some of the most frequent symptoms of depression are; sad mood, irritability, low self-esteem, low energy, and negative thoughts about oneself. The longer that the depressive symptoms persist the higher the risk of developing suicidal thoughts. Patients could be at a higher risk for suicide when the hopeless thoughts are very pervasive, or soon after they start to feel better from the depression and suddenly become more energetic, During this transition, people find the energy that they were lacking to fulfill their suicidal plans. It is very important when teens are started on antidepressant medication, to follow your doctor's recommendations and to report back any sudden changes in behavior, energy, or demeanor. In some patients with a family history of bipolar disorder, starting an antidepressant can be risky because they might be in a higher risk of developing a hypomanic episode. When we use antidepressants in this population, we always follow the patients closely and sometimes we combine antidepressants with mood stabilizers(4).

Bipolar Disorder and Suicide: Navigating the Peaks and Valleys of Emotion

Teens with bipolar disorder, find themselves navigating a roller coaster of emotional highs and lows—a journey marked by intense mood swings and unpredictable shifts in behavior. There is a heightened risk of suicide among teens with bipolar disorder, highlighting the impulsive and reckless tendencies that often accompany manic episodes. Is very important to follow treatment recommendations closely when supporting your teen with bipolar disorder, changes in the sleep pattern, mood, and substance abuse can trigger manic episodes and put patients at risk of suicide (7-8).

Anxiety Disorders and Suicide: Confronting the Shadows of Fear

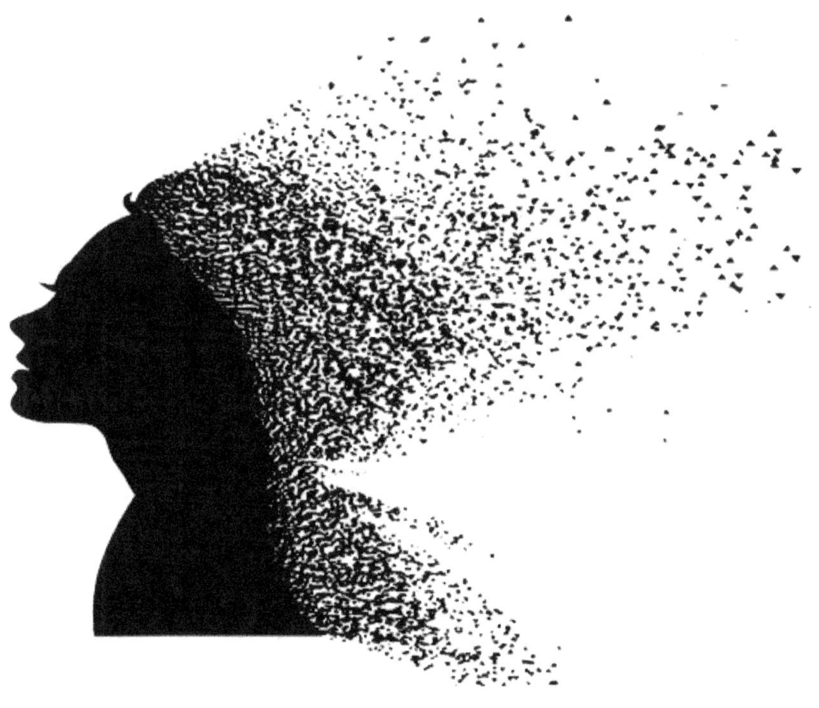

Anxiety disorders, with their insidious whispers of doubt and fear, cast a long shadow over the lives of teens—threatening to engulf them in a vortex of worry and despair (4). **Generalized Anxiety and Suicide: Drowning in a Sea of Worry**

For teens grappling with generalized anxiety disorder, each day becomes a relentless battle against a tide of worry and apprehension—a battle that can leave them feeling overwhelmed and exhausted. There is a heightened risk of suicide among teens with generalized anxiety disorder, secondary to the pervasive sense of uncertainty and dread that can accompany their symptoms. The combination of therapy and medication can help teens struggling with anxiety decreasing the risk of suicide.

Obsessive-Compulsive Disorder and Suicide: Trapped in a Cycle

of Fear

In the intricate web of obsessive-compulsive disorder, teens find themselves in a relentless cycle of intrusive thoughts and compulsive rituals—a cycle that threatens to consume them in a spiral of fear and anxiety. OCD poses some unique challenges about suicide risk among teens, there could be a profound sense of shame and isolation that can accompany their symptoms. Teens at times could struggle with suicidal obsessions, and like any obsession is a feeling that they don't want to have, but it keeps coming back to their minds. Working with a skilled therapist who teaches the teen coping strategies from cognitive behavioral therapy to manage their obsession could be helpful.

Panic Disorder and Suicide

Teens confront a relentless onslaught of terror and dread—a tidal wave of panic that threatens to overwhelm their senses and leave them gasping for air. Patients with panic disorder have an increased risk of suicide, perhaps because of the debilitating nature of panic attacks and the profound sense of helplessness that can accompany their symptoms. Some studies have identified increased symptoms of panic in some patients in the last 30 minutes before attempting suicide. There are effective pharmacologic treatments to improve the acute physical symptoms of panic, as well as relaxation techniques that can be helpful in managing the panic symptoms.

Post-Traumatic Stress Disorder and Suicide

For individuals coping with post-traumatic stress disorder (PTSD), each day becomes a relentless battle against the ghosts of the past—a battle marked by intrusive memories, flashbacks, and nightmares that threaten to engulf them in a sea of worry. Patients with PTSD frequently endorse suicidal thoughts, perhaps due to the pervasive sense of hopelessness, guilt, and shame that can accompany their symptoms.

LGBTQ and Suicide: Confronting the Shadows of Discrimination

and Stigma

In the terrain of LGBTQ mental health, individuals find themselves navigating a landscape marked by discrimination, stigma, and social rejection—a landscape that can leave them feeling isolated, marginalized, and invisible. LGBTQ teens face special unique challenges about suicide risk, there is a profound impact of minority stress, internalized homophobia, and rejection on their mental and emotional well-being. There are special challenges for transgender teens who feel uncomfortable with their gender and struggle to socially navigate a complicated, confusing reality. Having a supportive parent who accepts them as they are and supports them in their journey is a protective factor when considering suicide risk. Finding a supportive peer group is especially crucial in this population (4).

Substance Abuse and Suicide: Drowning in the Depths of Addiction

Teens who struggle with substance abuse are at higher risk for suicide. Perhaps as they confront a relentless cycle of dependency, withdrawal, and despair—a cycle that threatens to consume them in a spiral of addiction and self-destruction. For teens who are abusing drugs, each day becomes a relentless battle against the demons of dependency, withdrawal, and despair. Teens who are coping with addiction have a profound sense of emptiness and disconnection that can drive them to contemplate suicide as a means of escape from their pain and suffering.

By offering teens the support, validation, and resources they need to address their substance abuse issues, we can help them find hope and healing. With empathy and understanding as our guiding principles, we can empower teens to reclaim their lives and rewrite their stories with courage and resilience. Coping with a teen who is struggling with addiction, might have a tremendous impact on the family, seeking support in your community, for any specific substrate abuse treatment center close to you is paramount. Depending on the specific substance, and the degree of the addiction, some teens might need an inpatient detoxification before they can ever embark on the healing process. Getting a substance abuse evaluation early on will help the teen create the resources they need to be sober (19-20).

Kids in the Foster System/Adoption and Suicide: Navigating the Fragmented Landscape of Identity and Belonging

For kids in the foster system or adoption, each transition becomes a journey marked by uncertainty, instability, and loss—a journey that can leave them feeling hopeless, confused and longing. The profound impact of attachment disruptions, identity issues, and relational trauma on their mental and emotional well-being puts teens in the foster system at higher risk of suicide.

Conclusion: Cultivating Compassion and Understanding

Understanding the intricate interplay between mental illness and suicide is paramount. Behind every diagnosis lies a story—a story of resilience, courage, and unwavering determination to reclaim life in the face of adversity.

By fostering a culture of compassion, understanding, and support, we can empower individuals to navigate the darkest of nights and emerge into the dawn of a new day filled with hope, healing, and possibility. With empathy and compassion as our guides, may we walk alongside those who bear the weight of unseen wounds, offering solace and support in their moments of greatest need. As parents recognizing that we play an important role in helping our teens manage these symptoms is key. Asking for support when you as a parent need it is important and necessary.

8

Navigating Teen Suicide Risk: Understanding Warning Signs and Building Support

Recognizing the signs of suicide risk among teens is probably one of the most important steps that you can take as a parent. The signs might be different for each teen, is important to have an open and honest conversation with your teen so you can further understand, how to identify when they are at higher risk, so you can deploy all the help they will need at the moment.

Suicidal Ideation

At the heart of teen suicide risk lies the insidious whisper of suicidal ideation—a silent cry for help that can easily go unnoticed. Suicidal ideation among teens often serves as a silent cry for help—an expression of inner pain and despair that may go unnoticed or misunderstood. Is very important to recognize and validate the presence of suicidal thoughts, acknowledging the depth of emotional distress that teens may be experiencing (4).

For teens grappling with suicidal ideation, each thought becomes a heavy burden—an unwelcome companion that weighs upon their hearts and minds. It is very scary for teens at the beginning perhaps because of the stigma, to be open about their suicidal thoughts. When you hear from your teen that they are having suicidal thoughts, is always very important to take it seriously and always address it with compassion and understanding, offering teens a safe space to express their feelings and seek support (4).

Understanding the underlying triggers and motivations behind suicidal ideation is paramount of guiding effective intervention and support efforts. By fostering open communication and creating a supportive environment for teens to express their feelings, we can help them feel heard, valued, and understood. that behind every suicidal thought lies a complex web of emotions and experiences—a story waiting to be heard and validated with empathy and compassion. With attentive care and unwavering support, we can empower teens to navigate their darkest moments and find hope and healing on their journey toward recovery (21).

History of Self-Harming Behavior: Tracing the Scars of Pain

For teens with a history of self-harming behavior, each scar becomes a silent testament to the depths of their pain and suffering. Self-harm is an ineffective way of coping with severe distress. Teens who self-harm are at higher risk of suicide. Is very scary as a parent to discover that your teen has been self-harming. Teens will go to great lengths to hide their scars. The most important step is to identify the drivers of self-harm and work closely with your teen and a therapist to identify other healthy ways to cope with distress. Certain interventions are important to do at home, reducing access to any instruments that your teen is using for self-harm (knives, scissors, pins, box cutters). Supervise your teen closely, especially in moments of distress, and offer distraction, company, or anything that can help them keep their mind from hurting themselves(41).

Creating a supportive environment is foundational to preventing self-harm in adolescents. Hollander advocates for open communication and fostering trusting relationships where teens feel safe expressing their emotions without fear of judgment.

Education plays a pivotal role in equipping adolescents with healthy coping mechanisms and emotional regulation skills. Working closely with a therapist can teach teens alternative ways to manage distress and navigate difficult emotions constructively, DBT is one of the therapy techniques that have demonstrated effectiveness in teaching skills to decrease self-harm behavior (41).

Early intervention is key to addressing underlying issues contributing to self-harm tendencies. Is important to identify risk factors and provide timely access to mental health resources and support services (41).

Moreover, cultivating a culture of empathy and understanding helps diminish the stigma surrounding mental health struggles, encouraging adolescents to seek help when needed (41).

Goodbye Letters: The Final Farewell

Goodbye letters serve as poignant indicators of imminent danger in suicidal patients. Is important to recognize the significance of these letters as final expressions of despair and farewell. They often reflect a profound sense of hopelessness and emotional pain. Please take goodbye letters seriously, recognizing them as urgent calls for intervention. Understanding the depth of despair conveyed in these letters can guide compassionate and effective responses, offering support and connection to those who feel lost in their Darkest Moments.

Goodbye letters are signs of impending suicide, offering support and intervention before it's too late. If you found a goodbye letter, please make sure your teen is getting the appropriate level of care that they need, consider taking your teen to the emergency room if you feel you are unable to ensure their safety at the moment(7).

Disengagement: Drifting Away

In the quiet moments of disengagement, teens drift further from the world around them—a silent withdrawal that can signal deep-seated pain and isolation. When you observe disengagement in your teen, you should try to reach out and offer support to teens in need. At times it might be unwelcomed at the beginning, but later they will be grateful that you did. Teens might feel isolated, and lonely, is important to foster meaningful connections and support networks (4).

Low Self-Esteem: The Weight of Worthlessness

In the shadow of low self-esteem, teens struggle with feelings of worthlessness and inadequacy—a silent struggle that can impact their sense of self-worth and belonging. It is important to foster a culture of acceptance and validation, offering teens the support and encourage-ment they need to cultivate a positive self-image (4).

9

Supporting a Suicidal Teen: A Family's Compassionate Journey

In the intricate tapestry of family dynamics, navigating the challenges of a suicidal teen requires unwavering love, empathy, and understanding. As we embark on this journey of healing and support, it's essential to embrace proactive strategies that foster resilience and promote well-being.

1. Be There for Your Teen: The Power of Presence

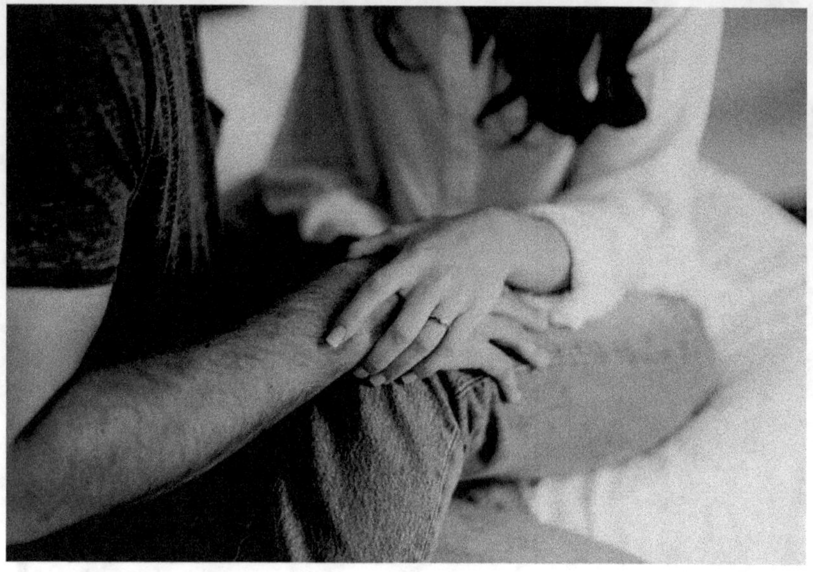

The simple act of being present can offer solace and reassurance to a struggling teen. Creating a safe and supportive environment where your teen feels heard, valued, and understood lays the foundation for healing and connection.

2. Assess the Risk: Understanding the Warning Signs

Vigilance is key in identifying the warning signs of suicide risk in teens. Pay attention to changes in behavior, mood swings, withdrawal from activities, and expressions of hopelessness or despair. Engage in open and honest conversations with your teen to gain insight into their emotional well-being and concerns(7).

3. Lethal Means Restriction: Creating a Safe Environment

Limiting access to lethal means, such as firearms, medications, or sharp objects, can prevent impulsive acts of self-harm or suicide. Secure potentially harmful items in the home and communicate openly with your teen about the importance of safety and well-being. If there is a firearm in your house, seriously consider for the time being (your teen being suicidal), removing the firearm from your house, if this is not possible then consider getting a password or fingerprint-protected gun safe, that is one of the most important life-saving interventions that you can do to help your teen who is currently struggling with suicidal thoughts (40).

4. Proactive Listening: Cultivating Empathy and Understanding

STOP

TALKING

AND

LISTEN

Effective communication lies at the heart of supporting a suicidal teen. Practice active listening, empathy, and validation, allowing your teen to express their feelings without judgment or criticism. Validate their experiences and emotions, offering support and reassurance along the way (4, 8).

5. When to Get Professional Help: Seeking Guidance and Support

Recognize the limitations of family support and know when to seek professional help. If your teen's symptoms persist or worsen, or if they express thoughts of suicide, it's crucial to consult mental health professionals or crisis intervention services immediately. Don't hesitate to reach out for guidance and support—it's a proactive step toward your teen's well-being. If everything fails, and the next available appointment to see a mental health professional is too far away, consider calling 988 or taking your teen to the nearest emergency room if you feel there are acute safety issues (if you feel they are not able to keep themselves safe). Or if they are not cooperating in creating a safety plan to prevent suicide.

Conclusion: Navigating the Journey with Compassion and Courage

Supporting a suicidal teen is a journey marked by compassion, resilience, and unwavering love. By embracing proactive strategies, fostering open communication, and seeking professional guidance when needed, families can provide the nurturing environment essential for their teen's healing and recovery. Together, let us embark on this journey with empathy and courage, offering hope and support to those who need it most.

10

Helping Your Teen Rediscover a Life Worth Living

As parents helping teens rediscover hope and purpose in life, is one of the most important legacies you can give to your teen. By incorporating practices like radical acceptance, positive thinking, and mindfulness, families can support their teens in building resilience and finding meaning in their journey toward healing.

Creating Hope:

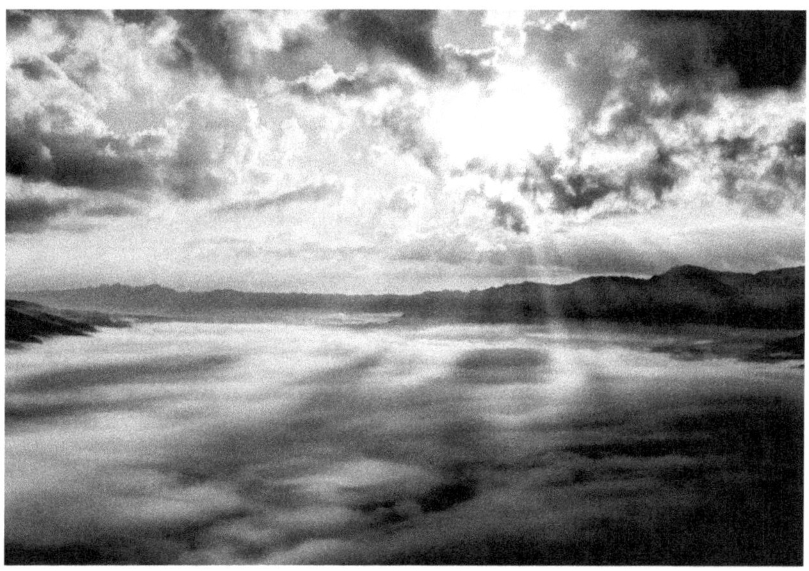

- ●Encourage your teen to envision a future filled with possibilities and potential.
- ●Foster a sense of optimism by highlighting past successes and moments of joy (you can use old pictures, old videos, old family memories).
- ●Remind your teen that hope is a powerful force that can guide them through even the darkest of times. Give them examples of things that you consider hopeful in your life and their life.
- ●Bring positive experiences, that help them see their potential
- ●Take a walk with your teen, in a place that you have never been before, and help them focus on all the positive things that surround you in the moment.

Discovering Hobbies:

- ●Explore activities and interests that bring joy and fulfillment to your teen's life.
- ●Encourage exploration and experimentation to find hobbies that resonate with their passions.
- ●Engage in activities together as a family to foster connection and shared experiences.
- Building Community Support:
- ●Connect your teen with supportive individuals and resources within the community.
- ●Seek out support groups, therapy programs, and peer networks that can offer encouragement and understanding.
- ●Encourage involvement in community service or volunteer opportunities to cultivate a sense of belonging and purpose.

Building Peer Support:

- ●Foster healthy friendships and connections with peers who uplift and support your teen.
- ●Encourage open communication and vulnerability in their relationships.
- ●Teach your teen the importance of setting boundaries and advocating for their well-being in their friendships.

Radical Acceptance:

- ●Embrace the concept of radical acceptance, acknowledging the reality of your teen's struggles without judgment or resistance. (4)
- ●Validate their experiences and emotions, allowing them to feel heard and understood. (4)

- ●Practice mindfulness techniques to cultivate a sense of peace and acceptance in the present moment. (4)
- Balancing Acceptance and Change:
- ●Help your teen find a balance between accepting their current circumstances and striving for positive change.
- ●Encourage small steps toward growth and healing, celebrating progress along the way.
- ●Remind your teen that change is a gradual process and setbacks are a natural part of the journey.

Positive Thinking:

- ●Cultivate a mindset of optimism and resilience in your teen.
- ●Encourage positive self-talk and affirmations to counter negative thought patterns.
- ●Help your teen reframe challenges as opportunities for growth and learning.

By cultivating an optimistic mindset, individuals can harness the power of positive thinking to navigate life's challenges with courage and hope. Seligman emphasizes the importance of reframing negative thoughts and embracing a perspective of optimism and gratitude. By focusing on strengths, achievements, and moments of joy, individuals can counteract feelings of despair and hopelessness that often precede suicidal ideation. Positive thinking fosters a sense of agency and empowerment, enabling individuals to envision a future filled with possibilities and potential. Through intentional practice and mindfulness, individuals can cultivate a resilient mindset that serves as a powerful buffer against the storms of life. In the journey of suicide prevention, positive thinking stands as a beacon of light, guiding individuals toward a path of healing, growth, and renewal. (42)

Relaxation Techniques:(44-45)

●Teach your teen relaxation techniques such as deep breathing, progressive muscle relaxation, and visualization.

●Encourage regular exercise and physical activity to reduce stress and promote overall well-being.

●Create a calming environment at home with soothing music, aromatherapy, or gentle lighting.

Mindfulness:(45)

●Practice mindfulness exercises with your teen to cultivate awareness and presence in the moment.

●Encourage mindful eating, walking, and listening as opportunities for connection and reflection.

●Explore guided meditation and mindfulness apps as tools for relaxation and self-discovery.

Searching for Meaning:

- ●Help your teen explore their values, passions, and sense of purpose in life.
- ●Encourage reflection and introspection to uncover what truly matters to them.
- ●Support your teen in setting meaningful goals and aspirations that align with their values and beliefs.

The work of Viktor Frankl on how we search for meaning can be helpful, in an attempt to think how we help teens search for meaning. The pursuit of meaning is intrinsic to the human condition, offering solace and purpose in the face of adversity. To prevent suicide, Frankl advocates for individuals to embark on an introspective journey of self-discovery, delving deep into the depths of their innermost desires and aspirations. By uncovering the unique meaning and purpose inherent in their lives, individuals can find renewed strength and resolve to confront life's challenges with courage and determination. Frankl's philosophy underscores the transformative power of meaning-making in suffering, offering a profound sense of connection and fulfillment that transcends the pain of existence. Through the search for meaning, individuals cultivate a resilient mindset that imbues their lives with purpose and significance, illuminating a path toward healing, hope, and renewal amidst the shadows of despair.

Building a Purposeful Future:(43)

- ●Assist your teen in setting realistic goals and creating a plan for achieving them.
- ●Foster a sense of agency and autonomy by involving your teen in decision-making processes.
- ●Encourage exploration of potential career paths, educational opportunities, and personal interests.

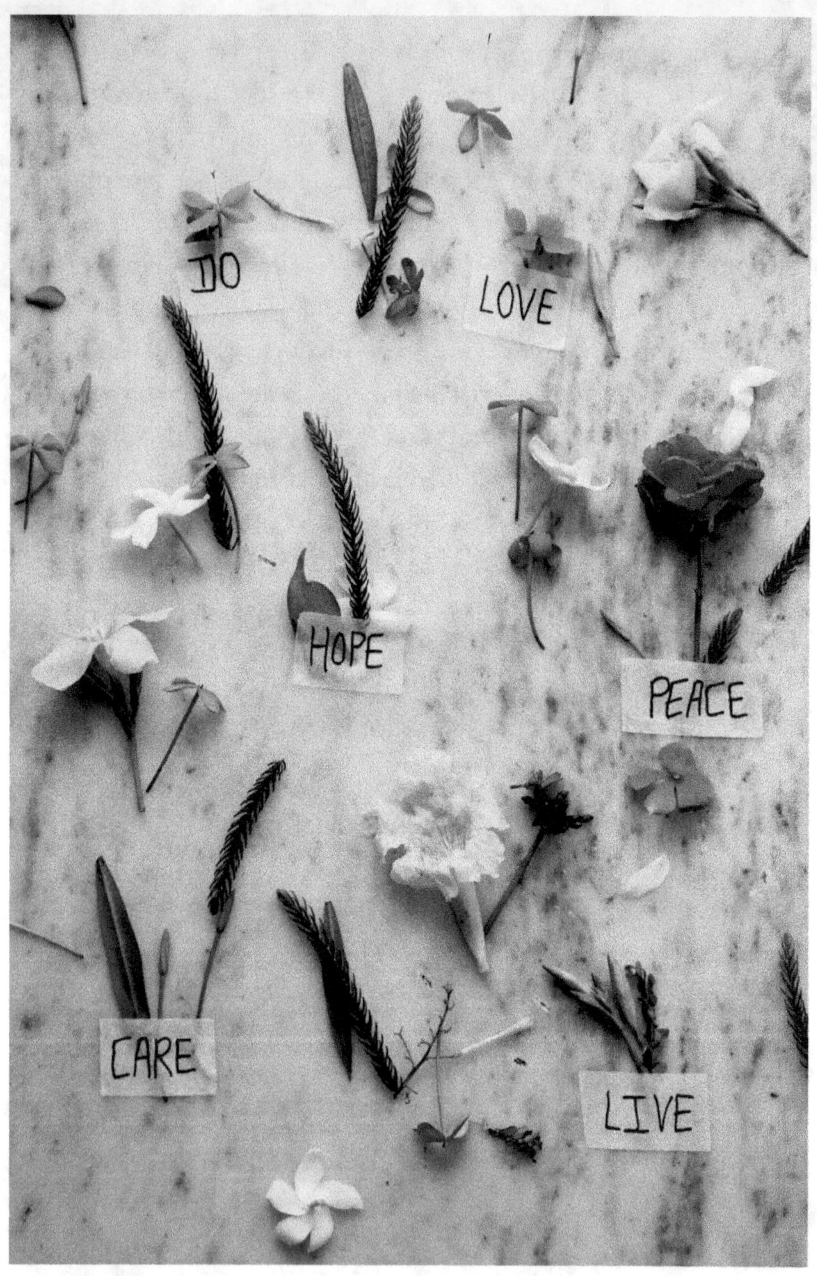
DO
LOVE
HOPE
PEACE
CARE
LIVE

•

Creating a Hope Box:(44)

- ●Assemble a collection of meaningful objects, photos, and mementos that inspire hope and joy.
- ●Encourage your teen to add items that evoke positive memories and feelings of gratitude.
- ●Use the hope box as a source of comfort and inspiration during difficult times.
- ●There is a great resource in the form of an app, the virtual hope box, that has great tools that can also be personalized to make it more meaningful for your teen, the app has a section on various relaxation techniques, some games for distraction, some quotes for encouragement, a phone that is a direct link to a suicide prevention line, coping card. Is such a great resource, please make sure your teen downloads the app on their phone.
- By incorporating these practices into your family's daily life, you can help your teen rediscover a life filled with hope, purpose, and meaning. With compassion, understanding, and unwavering support, you can empower your teen to embrace their journey of healing and rediscovery, one step at a time.

•

11

Final Thoughts on Teen Suicide Prevention: Nurturing Hope and Healing

It's crucial to acknowledge the pivotal role of caregivers in fostering resilience and promoting mental wellness for teens. As we reflect on the journey of suicide prevention, celebrating successes and fostering open lines of communication emerge as essential pillars in building a culture of support and understanding.

Helping the Caregiver: Nurturing Resilience and Compassion

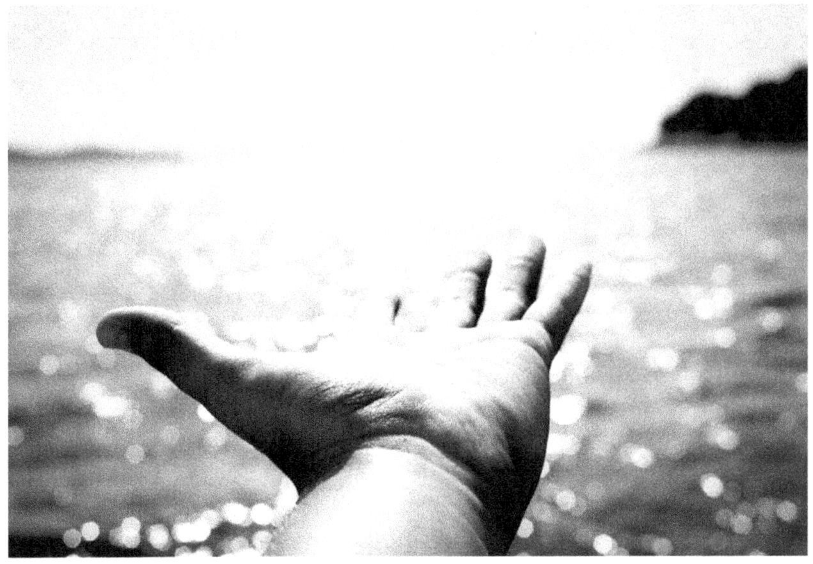

Caregivers play a pivotal role in the lives of teens struggling with suicidal thoughts and behaviors. It's imperative to provide caregivers with the support, resources, and guidance they need to navigate the complexities of teen mental health. From accessing therapy and support groups to practicing self-care and boundary-setting, caregivers must prioritize their well-being to effectively support their teens on their journey toward healing. Remember the old saying "You have to put on your oxygen mask before helping others". Unless you take care of your feelings is going to be hard to effectively be there for your teen (4).

Celebrating Success: Cultivating Resilience and Empowerment

In the journey of suicide prevention, every small victory is a cause for celebration. Whether it's reaching out for help, attending therapy sessions, or engaging in self-care activities, each step forward is a testament to resilience and strength. By celebrating successes, we validate the efforts of teens and caregivers alike, fostering a sense of empowerment and hope in the face of adversity.

Open Line of Communication: Fostering Connection and Understanding

Effective communication is the cornerstone of teen suicide prevention. Creating a safe and nonjudgmental space for teens to express their thoughts and feelings is paramount. Caregivers must prioritize active listening, empathy, and validation, allowing teens to feel heard, valued, and understood. By fostering open lines of communication, we bridge the gap between silence and understanding, nurturing connections that can save lives.

Building the Conversation about Mental Wellness: Embracing the Journey

The conversation about mental wellness must extend beyond crisis intervention to encompass an ongoing journey of self-discovery and growth. By destigmatizing mental health challenges and promoting a culture of acceptance and support, we create space for teens to explore their emotions, seek help when needed, and cultivate resilience in the face of adversity. Mental wellness becomes a shared journey, guided by compassion, understanding, and a commitment to nurturing the well-being of ourselves and those around us.

In conclusion, teen suicide prevention is not merely about saving lives—it's about fostering hope, healing, and resilience in the hearts and minds of our youth. By empowering caregivers, celebrating successes, fostering open communication, and embracing mental wellness as an ongoing journey, we can create a world where every teen feels valued, supported, and empowered to embrace life's challenges with courage and determination. Together, let us continue the conversation, nurture connections, and cultivate a future where every teen knows that hope is always within reach.

Thank you for taking the time to read this book, if you think it was helpful, I encourage you to leave a review so other parents can also learn about it.

12

References

1.https://newsroom.clevelandclinic.org/2023/03/01/cleveland-clinic-ranked-no-2-hospital-in-the-world-by-newsweek-3/

2.https://health.usnews.com/best-hospitals/area/oh/cleveland-clinic-6410670#overview

3. Brown, Brené, Daring Greatly: How the Courage to Be Vulnerable Transforms the Way We Live, Love, Parent, and Lead. New York, NY, Gotham Books, 2012.

4.Linehan, M. M. (2015). Building a life worth living. New York: Random House.

5.Falcone T, Janigro D, Lovell R, Simon B, Brown CA, Herrera M, Myint AM, Anand A. S100B blood levels and childhood trauma in adolescent inpatients. J Psychiatr Res. 2015 Mar;62:14-22. doi: 10.1016/j.jpsychires.2014.12.002. Epub 2014 Dec 25. PMID: 25669696; PMCID: PMC4413930.

6.Babcock L, Byczkowski T, Mookerjee S, Bazarian JJ. Ability of S100B to predict severity and cranial CT results in children with TBI. Brain Inj: [BI] 2012;26(11):1372–80

7.Jobes, D. A. (2023). Managing suicidal risk: A collaborative approach. Guilford Publications.

8.Linehan, M., M., (2014). DBT Training Manual. New York, NY: The Guilford Press.

9.McCauley E, Berk MS, Asarnow JR, Adrian M, Cohen J, Korslund K, Avina C, Hughes J, Harned M, Gallop R, Linehan MM. Efficacy of Dialectical Behavior Therapy for Adolescents at High Risk for Suicide: A Randomized Clinical Trial. JAMA Psychiatry. 2018 Aug 1;75(8):777-785. doi: 10.1001/jamapsychiatry.2018.1109. Erratum in: JAMA Psychiatry. 2018 Aug 1;75(8):867. PMID: 29926087; PMCID: PMC6584278.

10. Simpson SA, Goans CRR, Loh RM, Ryall KA, Middleton M, Dalton A. Use of an Agitation Measure to Screen for Suicide and Self-Harm Risk Among Emergency Department Patients. J Acad Consult Liaison Psychiatry. 2023 Jan-Feb;64(1):3-12. doi: 10.1016/j.jaclp.2022.07.004. Epub 2022 Jul 16. PMID: 35850464.

11. Rogers ML, Ringer FB, Joiner TE. A meta-analytic review of the association between agitation and suicide attempts. Clin Psychol Rev. 2016 Aug;48:1-6. doi: 10.1016/j.cpr.2016.06.002. Epub 2016 Jun 16. PMID: 27348187.

12. Hill RM, Kaplow JB, Oosterhoff B, Layne CM. Understanding grief reactions, thwarted belongingness, and suicide ideation in be-

reaved adolescents: Toward a unifying theory. J Clin Psychol. 2019 Apr;75(4):780-793. doi: 10.1002/jclp.22731. Epub 2019 Jan 12. PMID: 30636043.

13. . Franklin JC, Ribeiro JD, Fox KR, Bentley KH, Kleiman EM, Huang X, Musacchio KM, Jaroszewski AC, Chang BP,Nock MK. Risk factors for suicidal thoughts and behaviors: A meta-analysis of 50 years of research. Psychol Bull.2017;143(2):187-232.

14. Jobes DA, Eyman JR, Yufit RI. How clinicians assess suicide risk in adolescents and adults. Crisis Interv Time-L.1995;2(1):1-12.

15. Kothgassner OD, Goreis A, Robinson K,et al. Efficacy of dialectical behavior therapy for adolescent self-harm and suicidal ideation: a systematic review and meta-analysis. Psychol Med. 2021 May;51(7):1057-1067

16. Ougrin D, Tranah T, Stahl D, Moran P, Asarnow JR. Therapeutic interventions for suicide attempts and self-harm in adolescents: systematic review and meta-analysis. J Am Acad Child Adolesc Psychiatry. 2015 Feb;54(2):97-107.e2

17. Jobes DA. The collaborative assessment and management of suicidality (CAMS): An evolving evidence-based clinical approach to suicidal risk. Suicide Life Threat Behav. 2012;42(6):640-653.

18. O'Connor, S. S., Brausch, A., Anderson, A. R., & Jobes, D. A. (2014). Applying the
collaborative assessment and management of suicidality (CAMS) to suicidal adolescents. International Journal of- Behavioral Consultation and Therapy, 9, 53-58.

19. Nordentoft, M. (2016). Effectiveness of dialectical behavior therapy versus collaborative assessment andmangament of suicidality treatment for reduction of self-harm in adults with borderline personality traits anddisorder - A randomized observer-blinded clinical trial. Depression and Anxiety, 33, 520–530.

20. Swift JK, Trusty WT, Penix EA. The effectiveness of the Collaborative Assessment and Management of Suicidality (CAMS) compared to alternative treatment conditions: A meta-analysis. Suicide Life Threat Behav. 2021 Oct;51(5):882-896. doi: 10.1111/sltb.12765. Epub 2021 May 17. PMID: 33998028.

21. Adrian M, Blossom JB, Chu PV, Jobes D, McCauley E. Collaborative Assessment and Management of Suicidality for Teens: A Promising Frontline Intervention for Addressing Adolescent Suicidality. Pract Innov (Wash D C). 2021 Aug 26;7(2):154-167. doi: 10.1037/pri0000156. PMID: 35747427; PMCID: PMC9211019.

22. .Falcone T. First randomized trial of ketamine for youth suicidality to launch with NIH support. Consult QD. 10/2020https://consultqd.clevelandclinic.org/first-randomized-trial-of-ketamine-for-youth-suicidality-to-launch-with-nih-support/

23. Falcone T. Podcast Neuropathways. Suicidality in Individuals with neurologic disorders https://podcasts.apple.com/us/podcast/effect-of-adverse-childhood-experiences/id1467738002?i=1000525595410

24. Ciccone A. Integration of Mental Health screening may prevent suicide in epilepsy 12/6/15 Neurology advisor https://www.neurologyadvisor.com/conference-highlights/aes-2015/integration-of-mental-health-screening-may-prevent-suicide-in-epilepsy/

25. OpenAI. (2024). ChatGPT (3.5) [Large language model]. https://chat.openai.com

26. Wolfelt, A. D. (2003). Understanding your grief: ten essential touchstones for finding hope and healing your heart. Companion Press.

27. Haig M.(2016) Reasons to Stay Alive . Penguin Books.

28. Sander LB, Beisemann M, Doebler P, Micklitz HM, Kerkhof A, Cuijpers P, Batterham P, Calear A, Christensen H, De Jaegere E, Domhardt M, Erlangsen A, Eylem-van Bergeijk O, Hill R, Mühlmann C, Österle M, Pettit J, Portzky G, Steubl L, van Spijker B, Tighe J, Werner-Seidler A, Büscher R. The Effects of Internet-Based Cognitive Behavioral Therapy for Suicidal Ideation or Behaviors on Depression, Anxiety, and Hopelessness in Individuals With Suicidal Ideation: Systematic Review and Meta-Analysis of Individual Participant Data. J Med Internet Res. 2023 Jun 26;25:e46771. doi: 10.2196/46771. PMID: 37358893; PMCID: PMC10337381.

29. Plioplys S, Dunn DW, Caplan R. 10-year research update review: psychiatric problems in children with epilepsy. Journal of the American Academy of Child & Adolescent Psychiatry. 2007 Nov;46(11):1389-402.

30. Jones JE, Watson R, Sheth R, Caplan R, Koehn M, Seidenberg M, et al. Psychiatric comorbidity in children with new onset epilepsy. Developmental Medicine & Child Neurology. 2007 Jul;49(7):493-7.

31. Silveira,D.,Mishra,L.,Franco,E.,Tesar,G.,Janigro,D.,Falcone,T. Depression and Epilepsy in children. Epilepsia. 2008;49(7).

32. Plioplys S. Depression in children and adolescents with epilepsy.

Epilepsy Behav. 2003 Oct;4(Suppl 3):S39-45.

33. Caplan R, Gillberg C, Dunn DW, Spence SJ. Psychiatric Disorders In Children. In: Engel J, Pedley TA, editors. Epilepsy A comprehensive textbook. 2nd ed. Philadelphia, PA: Lippincott Williams & Wilkins; 2008. p. 2179-93.

34. Falcone T, Dagar A, Castilla-Puentes RC, Anand A, Brethenoux C, Valleta LG, Furey P, Timmons-Mitchell J, Pestana-Knight E. Digital conversations about suicide among teenagers and adults with epilepsy: A big-data, machine learning analysis. Epilepsia. 2020 May;61(5):951-958. doi: 10.1111/epi.16507. Epub 2020 May 8. PMID: 32383797; PMCID: PMC7384181.

35. Majidi S, O'Donnell HK, Stanek K, Youngkin E, Gomer T, Driscoll KA. Suicide Risk Assessment in Youth and Young Adults With Type 1 Diabetes. Diabetes Care. 2020 Feb;43(2):343-348. doi: 10.2337/dc19-0831. Epub 2019 Dec 10. PMID: 31822488; PMCID: PMC6971783.

36. Matlock KA, Yayah Jones NH, Corathers SD, Kichler JC. Clinical and psychosocial factors associated with suicidal ideation in adolescents with type 1 diabetes. J Adolesc Health 2017;61:471–47

37. Greydanus D, Patel D, Pratt H. Suicide risk in adolescents with chronic illness: implications for primary care and specialty pediatric practice: a review. Dev Med Child Neurol. 2010 Dec;52(12):1083-7. doi: 10.1111/j.1469-8749.2010.03771.x. Epub 2010 Aug 31. PMID: 20813018.

38. Ferro MA, Rhodes AE, Kimber M, Duncan L, Boyle MH, Georgiades K, Gonzalez A, MacMillan HL. Suicidal Behaviour Among Adolescents

and Young Adults with Self-Reported Chronic Illness. Can J Psychiatry. 2017 Dec;62(12):845-853. doi: 10.1177/0706743717727242. Epub 2017 Aug 17. PMID: 28814100; PMCID: PMC5714119.

39. Michalek IM, Caetano Dos Santos FL, Wojciechowska U, Didkowska J. Suicide risk among adolescents and young adults after cancer diagnosis: analysis of 34 cancer groups from 2009 to 2019. J Cancer Surviv. 2023 Jun;17(3):657-662. doi: 10.1007/s11764-023-01358-5. Epub 2023 Mar 17. PMID: 36930435; PMCID: PMC10209251.

40. Stanley, B., & Brown, G. (2012). Safety Planning Intervention: A brief intervention to mitigate suicide risk. Cognitive and Behavioral Practice, 19(2), 256–264.

41. Hollander M. (2017) Helping teens who cut, Using DBT skills to end self injury. The Guildford Press. Second Edition. Pgs 1-238

42. Seligman, M. E. P. (2006). Learned optimism: how to change your mind and your life. 1st Vintage Books ed. New York, NY, Vintage Books.

43. Frankl, V. E. (1992). Man's search for meaning: An introduction to logotherapy (4th ed.)

44. https://apps.apple.com/au/app/virtual-hope-box/id825099621

45. https://apps.apple.com/us/app/mindful-moments-by-ccw/id1449898637

46. Falcone T Telemedicine as a tool for suicide assessment in the time of COVID-19J Am Acad Child Adolesc Psychiatry. 2020 Oct; 59(10): S125.

REFERENCES

Published online 2020 Oct 16. doi: 10.1016/j.jaac.2020.07.486PMCID: PMC7567450

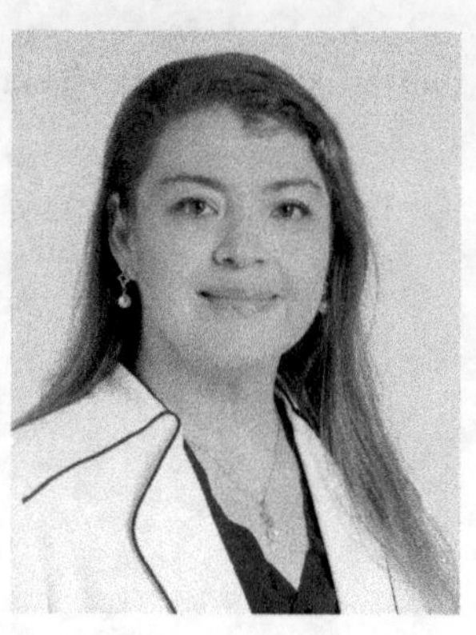

About the Author

Dr. Falcone is a child psychiatrist at Cleveland Clinic and assistant professor of Psychiatry and Neurology at Cleveland Clinic Lerner College of Medicine of Case Western Reserve University; She is a Clinician Scientist, which means that spends 50% of the time treating patients, 50% of the time doing research in suicide prevention. Dr. Falcone was CHIPS fellow, a Public Psychiatry Fellow, and APA leadership fellow. She was recognized as teacher of the year at Cleveland Clinic in 2007 and 2010. For the last 13 years she has been founded by HRSA, SAMHSA and NIMH, to improve the care for children with chronic medical illness (epilepsy) Project COPE, Project CARE and Project IMPACTT, She is also researching suicide prevention and interventions to improve treatments provided for youth at risk of suicide

You can connect with me on:

🌐 https://my.clevelandclinic.org/staff/8196-tatiana-falcone

Also by Tatiana Falcone

73

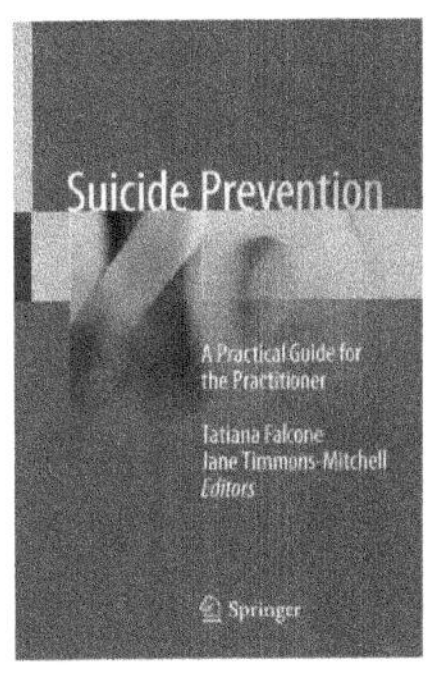

Suicide Prevention a Practical guide for the Practitioner

A guide to help clinicians manage suicidal patients in different settings.